THE ULTIMATE DIABETES COOKBOOK

Quick and Healthy Diabetes Recipes For Type 1 and Type 2 Diabetics

2nd Edition

Thomas James Williams

ISBN-: 9781070918204

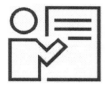

Diabetes is a group of diseases that result in too much sugar in the blood, in other words: high blood glucose. Also known as diabetes mellitus and sugar diabetes.

Diabetes means 'to syphon' in Greek and seems to first have been used around 250B.C. The word reflects the thirst manifested by sufferers. Aretaeus, the ancient Greek physician became aware of how copiously the afflicted passed urine. Much later in 1674, Thomas Willis, King Charles II's personal physician coined *Diabetes mellitus* by adding the Latin word for honey, finding as he had that a diabetic's urine seemed infused with honey and sugar.

As was the norm back in the 19th century, treatment for diabetes ranged from prescribing opium to bleeding and severe calorie-restricted diets, often as severe as tantamount to starvation. In 1889 German physicians linked the pancreas gland to diabetes which was quite the breakthrough in the puzzle. Dr. Frederick Banting succeeded remarkably in the challenge to isolate the pancreatic extract (insulin) by 1921. The first human received insulin treatment in January 1922. He went on to live to 27, after 13 years of ever-improving treatment. Banting won a Nobel Prize for his discovery.

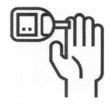

So we now know that peculiarly high levels of sugar or glucose in the blood is characteristic of diabetes, but what is the cause? And why do some people suffer from the condition and others not?

Levels of glucose in the blood increase, usually after eating, which activates the pancreas to release the hormone insulin. It is insulin's job to stimulate the muscle and fat cells to get the glucose out of the blood stream, and to stimulate the liver to metabolize the glucose. This activity regulates the levels of blood sugar. Diabetics, however, retain their high blood sugar levels, either due to ineffective or insufficient insulin or, or a lack of production of insulin. Let's simplify:

We can regard insulin as the **hormone of plenty**, released when glucose is plentiful. Insulin stimulates:

- fat cells and muscle to remove glucose from the blood

- adipose tissue to stockpile fat for energy reserves in the long term in the form of glucose

- cells to break glucose down and release energy as ATP

- cells to utilize glucose for protein synthesis

TYPE 1 AND TYPE 2 DIABETES

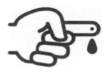

Forms of diabetes are:

Type 2 diabetes is a chronic condition linked to obesity that affects the way the body processes glucose.

Type 1 diabetes which is an autoimmune disorder and a chronic condition characterized by the pancreas producing too little or no insulin.

Gestational diabetes affects only pregnant women and is a form of high blood sugar.

Prediabetes is a condition in which blood sugar is high, although too low to be type 2 diabetes.

The symptoms of both the first two type of diabetes are similar and include:

- ℞ Excessive thirst/dry mouth

- ℞ Frequent urination

- ℞ Tingling or numbness in hands and feet

- ℞ Blurred vision

- ℞ Lack of energy/lethargy/tiredness

- Slow healing wounds

- Recurrent skin infections

Type 1 Diabetes

Approximately 10% of diabetics have type 1 diabetes, which is caused by an autoimmune reaction in which the body attacks those cells that produce insulin. The causes are genetic and environmental, resulting in very little or no insulin produced. It is most common in children or young adults. Treatment involves controlling blood glucose levels through daily injections of insulin. Nutritious eating and regular exercise should be part of the daily regime for managing type 1 diabetes.

Type 2 Diabetes

Of these diabetes types, type 2 diabetes is the most common, making up approximately 90% of all cases. Generally characterized by insulin resistance, the type 2 sufferer does not respond effectively to insulin which means continuously rising blood glucose levels and the resultant increased insulin production. Hyperglycaemia often follows when the pancreas is eventually exhausted, leaving diminished insulin production and consequentially higher blood sugar levels. Where type 2 used to be prevalent among adults, rising obesity occurrence, poor diet, urbanization, and sedentary lifestyles has resulted in its manifestation in children, teenagers and young adults.

Risk factors include:

- Family history of diabetes

- Overweight

- Sedentary lifestyle

- High blood pressure

- Ethnicity

- Age

- Diet

- History of gestational diabetes

- Poor nutrition while pregnant

- Impaired glucose tolerance (IGT) which involves higher than normal blood glucose, below the threshold for diabetes, but usually precedes onset of diabetes.

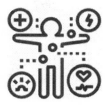

Factors most associated with the onset of type 2 diabetes are those lifestyle activities generally connected with urbanisation. It is believed that as many as 80% of type 2 diabetes cases could be pre-empted with regular physical activity and a healthy diet.

Effective regular physical activity means reducing sedentary time and combining resistance training with aerobic exercise.

What is considered a healthy diet?

- Reduced calorie intake in overweight individuals

- Replace saturated fats with unsaturated

- Include dietary fibre

- Don't smoke

- Don't drink

- Avoid added sugar

Sugar and hidden sugars are taboo on a diabetic diet. It is possible to reverse the condition and to manage it with a healthy eating routine.

℞ Drink water, tea or coffee rather than sugar sweetened beverages, fruit juice, or soda

℞ Eat poultry, lean cuts of white meat, or seafood rather than processed/red meat

℞ Alcoholic beverages to be limited to two a day

℞ Snack on nuts, fresh fruit, or yoghurt

℞ Eat green leafy vegetables, incorporating a minimum of three daily servings of vegetables

℞ Eat three daily servings or less of fresh fruit

℞ Rather than chocolate or jam, go with peanut butter

℞ Go with whole-grain pasta, bread, or rice rather than the white options

☙ Unsaturated fats are good, such as olive oil/canola oil/corn oil/ sunflower oil. Saturated fats are bad, such as coconut/palm oil, animal fat, butter, and ghee.

Low Glycaemic Diet

uses the Glycaemic Index (GI) to rank food that contains carbohydrates. The three GI ratings are low (55 or less), medium (56–69), and high (70 or more). Low-GI foods are digested and absorbed in a way that has less effect on blood sugar levels. Foods with high GI values get digested and absorbed quicker causing blood sugar levels to rise and fall dramatically.

The low-GI diet requires replacing high-GI foods with low-GI options. As such, we will outline the good and the bad and the preferred among them.

Low-GI foods:

- ○ **Fruit**: apples, pears, strawberries, peaches, apricots, plums, kiwi fruit

- ○ **Vegetables**: cauliflower, broccoli, carrots, celery, courgettes, tomatoes

- ○ **Starchy vegetables**: orange-fleshed sweet potatoes, yams, corn

- ○ **Dairy**: milk, yogurt, cheese, custard, almond milk, soymilk

- ○ **Grains**: pearl couscous, quinoa, barley, freekeh, buckwheat, semolina

- ○ **Bread**: whole grain, sourdough, multigrain, rye

- ○ **Cereals**: rolled oats, muesli, All-Bran

- ○ **Legumes**: baked beans, chickpeas, lentils, butter beans, kidney beans

- ○ **Pasta**: vermicelli, rice noodles

- ○ **Rice**: long-grain, brown rice, Basmati

No GI value/carbohydrate-free:

- ○ Meat

- ○ Eggs

- ○ Fish and seafood

- ○ Herbs and spices

- ○ Nuts

- ○ Fats and oils

Avoid these foods:

Bread: white bread, naan bread, bagels, Turkish/Lebanese bread, baguettes

Cereals: Rice Krispies, Froot Loops, Instant oats, Corn Flakes, Cocoa Krispies

Starchy vegetables: instant mashed potato

Pasta: instant noodles, corn pasta

Rice: medium-grain white rice, Jasmine, Calrose

Dairy: Rice milk, oat milk

Fruit: Watermelon

Savoury snacks: rice cakes, rice crackers, pretzels, corn chips

Cakes and biscuits: doughnuts, scones, cupcakes, waffles

Miscellaneous: liquorice, jellybeans, energy drinks

Suggestions:

- Unprocessed food usually has a lower glycaemic index than processed alternatives, so whole what bread is preferred to white bread

- Combining low-glycaemic and high-glycaemic foods counter the bad effects of high GI foods, and blood sugar rises slower

- Al-dente pasta has a lower GI than well done pasta

- High-fibre foods typically take longer to digest, raising blood sugar slowly

- When dining out, select low GI dishes with non-starchy veggies

- Limit high-glycaemic foods to small portions

- Whole grains are better so go with 100% whole grain toast rather than white bread

The Diabetes Plate Method

uses an easy formula to encourage more healthy food and less un-
healthy foods. The diet controls portion sizes of starchy, carbohydrates
which impact blood glucose levels and emphasises non-starchy vegetables, low in carbohydrate and rich in fibre, vitamins, and minerals.
Lean protein is also incorporated. The formula simply requires filling
half a standard size plate with non-starchy vegetables, one quarter
with starchy or whole grain foods and a quarter with lean proteins.
Fruit and low-fat dairy are allowed on the side, as are healthful fats
for food preparation.

RECIPES

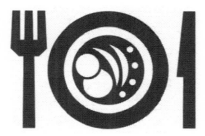

Regardless of what you're eating, diabetics should measure blood glucose before eating and two hours afterwards to determine the effect of meals. Morning fasting blood sugar may be affected by many factors, including stress, poor quality of sleep, or inadequate medication. Do no skip breakfast, and always try for a healthy option that'll help manage blood sugar levels.

BREAKFAST

Time: 2 mins | Serves 1

Calories: 404	Carbs: 38g	Fibre: 15.5g	Sugars: 16g	Protein: 12g

INGREDIENTS:

- ½ cup frozen blueberries
- ⅓ cup frozen strawberries
- 100g berry yogurt
- ¾ cup unsweetened almond milk
- ½ avocado
- 1 tsp flaxseed
- 1 handful spinach
- 1 tbsp chia seeds
- 4 ice cubes
- 1 scoop protein powder

PREPARATION:

1. Blend all the ingredients and enjoy

Time: 30 mins | Serves 4

Calories: 88	Carbs: 20g	Fibre: 0.6g	Sugars: 1.3g	Protein: 10g

INGREDIENTS:

♦ 12 slices lean turkey bacon

♦ 500g egg white

♦ 3 eggs

♦ 70g lean turkey sausage, chopped

♦ 70g chopped red bell pepper

♦ 70g finely chopped onion

♦ 70g baby spinach

♦ ½ finely chopped jalapeno chili,

♦ 1 finely chopped clove garlic

♦ If you want to use salt and pepper, do it

PREPARATION:

1. Heat oven to 351°F (180°C) and spray non-stick spray on muffin pan

2. Line inside of each muffin form with a slice of bacon and place a bit of spinach in each

3. Sauté onions, jalapeno, and garlic until the onions are translucent

4. Divide onion mix evenly between the 12 muffin forms, on top of spinach

5. Add chopped sausage and bell pepper to muffin forms

6. Whisk egg whites, eggs, salt and pepper together in mixing bowl

7. Cover veggies in muffin form with the egg mixture and bake on idle rack for 25 mins.

Time: 10 mins | Serves 2

Calories: 182	Carbs: 16.6g	Fibre: 2.3g	Sugars: 2.4g	Protein: 22.2g

INGREDIENTS:

- ♦ non-stick spray
- ♦ 40g raw oats
- ♦ 28g blueberries
- ♦ 1 scoop vanilla protein powder
- ♦ 3 (130g) egg whites
- ♦ ½ tsp baking powder
- ♦ 1 tbsp artificial sweetener
- ♦ ¼ cup water

PREPARATION:

1. Spray non-stick spray on pan and heat on stove at medium heat
2. Blend together all remaining ingredients
3. Pour batter evenly into heated pan to cover base with a thin layer
4. Cook for about 1 min on each side until fully cooked
5. Fresh berries are a suggestion for serving

Time: 10 mins | Serves 1

Calories: 266	Carbs: 18.8g	Fibre: 5.6g	Sugars: 11.6g	Protein: 17.8g

INGREDIENTS:

- ½ cup cottage cheese
- ¼ cup blackberries
- ¼ pomegranate, seeds removed
- 30g hazelnuts
- 14g coconut flakes, unsweetened

PREPARATION:

1. Pulse cottage cheese to a smooth and creamy consistency, about 2 to 3 mins

2. Over medium heat, toast hazelnuts and coconut flakes in a skillet for 2 to 3 mins. You might want to stir during heating

3. You decide when you want to eat it.

Time: 10 mins | Serves 1

| Calories: 291 | Carbs: 17.8g | Fibre: 6.7g | Sugars: 3g | Protein: 24g |

INGREDIENTS:

- ◆ 1 20cm tortilla
- ◆ 55g smoked salmon
- ◆ 2 tsp cream cheese
- ◆ 35g finely sliced red onion
- ◆ arugula
- ◆ pinch fresh basil and pepper

PREPARATION:

1. Warm tortilla in oven/microwave

2. Combine cream cheese, basil and pepper, and spread onto tortilla, topping with salmon, onion and arugula

3. Wrap and snack.

Time: 6 mins | Serves 1

Calories: 331	Carbs: 46g

INGREDIENTS:

- ½ cup rolled oats, cooked in ¼ cup milk and 3/4 cup water
- ½ medium apple, chopped
- 2 tbsp chopped unsalted almonds
- ground cinnamon

PREPARATION:

1. Cook the oats and serve sprinkled with the apple, nuts and cinnamon.

Time: 5 mins | Serves 1

Calories: 271	Carbs: 18g	Fibre: 5g	Sugars: 2g	Protein: 11g

INGREDIENTS:

- ◆ 1 slice toasted whole-wheat bread
- ◆ 1 fried egg
- ◆ ¼ avocado
- ◆ pinch garlic powder and pepper

PREPARATION:

1. Mash garlic powder, avocado, and pepper together

2. Add avo mix to toast with the fried egg

3. Serve and enjoy

TIME: 5 MINS | SERVES 1

Calories: 196	Carbs: 25g	Fibre: 2g	Sugars: 20g	Protein: 24g

INGREDIENTS:

- ♦ 1 cup Greek yogurt
- ♦ ½ cup blueberries
- ♦ 1 tsp honey

PREPARATION:

1. Serve yoghurt topped with blueberries and a drizzle of hone

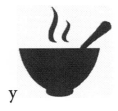

y

TIME: 7 MINS | SERVES 1

Calories: 317	Carbs: 7g	Fibre: 1g	Sugars: 5g	Protein: 22g

INGREDIENTS:

- ♦ whites of 2 eggs (ta-da)
- ♦ 1 tbsp milk
- ♦ 1 cup veg (mushrooms, tomatoes, onions, capsicum)
- ♦ 1 tbsp olive oil
- ♦ If you want to use salt and pepper, do it

PREPARATION:

1. Heat non-stick pan and add spoonful olive oil

2. Combine egg whites, salt, pepper and veggies with a spoonful of milk

3. Add to heated pan, spreading mixture evenly and cook through

4. Serve hot

Time: 20 mins | Serves 4

Calories: 247	Carbs: 36.7g	Fibre: 5.6g	Protein: 5.5g

INGREDIENTS:

- ♦ 100g oats porridge
- ♦ 50g bran flakes, crushed
- ♦ 1 tbsp agave nectar
- ♦ ½ tbsp olive oil
- ♦ 25g roughly chopped almonds
- ♦ 1½ tbsp honey

PREPARATION:

1. Preheat oven to320°F (160°C) and cover baking tray with baking parchment

2. Combine crushed bran, oats and almonds

3. Combine remaining ingredients and get to a temperature where it bubbles (boil) for 2 mins. Stir until a syrup consistency

4. Pour syrup over muesli and mix well

5. Spread muesli on prepared baking tray. Bake for 16 mins, stirring every 5 mins

6. Take it out of the heated environment before it dries out and allow to cool before storing in airtight container.

TIME: 7 MINS | SERVES 4

Calories: 430	Carbs: 0.8g	Fibre: 0g	Protein: 20.8g

INGREDIENTS:

- 4 eggs
- 400g thinly sliced pork sausage
- 2½ tbsp milk
- ½ tbsp olive oil

PREPARATION:

1. Brown sausage for 3 to 4 mins in heated oil over medium heat

2. Whisk milk and eggs together and add to the sausage in griddle pan. Cook through.

3. Serve immediately.

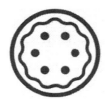

Time: 70 mins | Serves 4

Calories: 162	Carbs: 2.2g	Fibre: 0g	Protein: 13.5g

INGREDIENTS:

- ♦ 8 skewers
- ♦ 300g cooked tiger/king prawns
- ♦ 2⅞ tbsp olive oil
- ♦ 1⅞ tbsp sweet chilli sauce
- ♦ juice of 1 lemon
- ♦ tbsp Dijon mustard

PREPARATION:

1. For marinade, thoroughly mix olive oil, Dijon mustard, lemon juice and sweet chilli sauce

2. Add prawns and thoroughly coat in marinade

3. Refrigerate overnight, or at least for 1 hour

4. Skewer the prawns and grill for 5 mins until beginning to caramelise.

Time: 12 mins | Serves 4

Calories: 760	Carbs: 77g	Fibre: 5g	Protein: 60g

INGREDIENTS:

- ◆ 800g lamb cut, sliced
- ◆ 1⅛ tbsp vegetable oil
- ◆ 1 tbsp peeled ginger, chopped
- ◆ 4 garlic cloves, finely chopped
- ◆ 1 tbsp dark soy sauce
- ◆ 1 thinly sliced red chilli
- ◆ 300g fungi commonly called mushrooms, finely sliced
- ◆ 2⅞ to 3 sliced spring onions
- ◆ 800g cooked soba noodles, drained

PREPARATION:

1. Stir fry lamb, garlic, ginger, and chilli for 5 to 7 mins in oil heated in a wok until lamb browns

2. Add mushrooms and spring onions, fry for 3 mins

3. Add soy sauce and mix thoroughly

4. Serve with soba noodles.

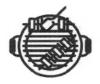

Time: 50 mins | Serves 4

Calories: 282	Carbs: 2g	Fibre: 2g	Protein: 18g

INGREDIENTS:

- 6 chicken drumsticks, skin on
- 120g ground almonds
- ½ tsp each ginger powder, dried parsley,
- dried sage, dried basil & mustard powder
- ¼ tsp Chinese five spice
- 2 tbsp olive oil
- 1 tsp paprika
- salt and ground black pepper
- ¼ tsp chili powder

PREPARATION:

1. Preheat oven to 370°F (181°C) and oil bottom of baking dish with olive oil

2. Shake spices, herbs and ground almonds in a plastic bag to mix

3. Pop chicken drumsticks into bag, shake, and rub mixture into chicken

4. Bake the chicken in the baking dish for 45 mins, turning 2 or 3 times to ensure even coating.

TIME: 5 MINS | SERVES 4

Calories: 179	Carbs: 13g	Fibre: 9g	Protein: 15.6g

INGREDIENTS:

- ◆ 150g spinach leaves
- ◆ 150g watercress, without stalks
- ◆ 2 grated carrots
- ◆ 100g halved cherry tomatoes
- ◆ 1 small red bell pepper, finely sliced
- ◆ 2 tbsp sunflower seeds, slightly toasted
- ◆ 100g tinned chickpeas, drained
- ◆ 100g feta cheese

PREPARATION:

1. Combine spinach, watercress, rocket, and grated carrots in a large bowl

2. Add cherry tomatoes and red bell pepper and combine all with sunflower seeds and chickpeas

3. Serve with feta and seasoning.

TIME: 20 MINS | SERVES 4

| Calories: 147 | Carbs: 19g | Fibre: 5g | Protein: 3.8g |

INGREDIENTS:

- ◆ 2 yellow peppers and 2 red peppers, cored and sliced thinly
- ◆ ½ baby marrow, chopped
- ◆ 2 peeled red onions, sliced thinly
- ◆ 400g tinned love fruit
- ◆ 4 cloves of garlic, peeled and crushed
- ◆ 2 tbsp olive oil
- ◆ salt and pepper to taste

PREPARATION:

1. Cook red onions and garlic in olive oil heated over medium heat until softened, approximately 3 to 4 mins

2. Add peppers and season to taste

3. Add tomatoes and cook covered for 15 mins

4. Serve warm

Time: 10 mins | Serves 2

Calories: 175	Carbs: 9.1g	Fibre: 0.8g	Protein: 13g

INGREDIENTS:

- 150g cubed salmon fillet
- 100g cubed halibut fillet
- 100g cubed tuna fillet
- 1 egg
- Soak a ½ stale wholegrain bread roll in water
- ½ bunch spring onions
- 2 sticks celery
- 1 carrot
- 1 tsp cornflour
- 300g seasonal vegetables, cut into pieces
- 2 tbsp sour cream (not fresh)
- 2 tbsp rapeseed oil
- 125 ml veg stock
- 1 tbsp chopped herbs
- 1 chilli
- If you want to use salt and pepper, do it

PREPARATION:

1. Mix fish, diced vegetables, egg and corn flour
2. Squeeze liquid out soaked roll and add to mixture
3. Season to taste, cover and set one side

4. Fry seasonal vegetables in half the rapeseed oil and add vegetables stock, season to taste

5. Stir sour cream and herbs into stock mixture before serving

6. Slowly fry fish mixture shaped into burgers in remaining heated rapeseed oil until both sides are golden brown

7. Serve seasonal vegetables topped with fish cakes.

Time: 50 mins | Serves 2

Calories: 312	Carbs: 35g	Fibre: 9g	Protein: 6.2g

INGREDIENTS:

- ◆ 1-1.25kg ripe tomatoes, quartered
- ◆ 2 chopped celery sticks
- ◆ 1 chopped onion
- ◆ 2 garlic cloves
- ◆ 1 chopped carrot
- ◆ 2 tsp tomato purée
- ◆ 2 bay leaves
- ◆ 2 tbsp olive oil
- ◆ 1200ml hot veg stock

PREPARATION:

1. Gently cook celery, onion, garlic, and carrot in heated olive oil over low heat for 10 mins

2. Add tomato purée, black pepper and tomatoes and then bay leaves. Simmer, stirring frequently over low heat for 10 mins

3. Pour hot stock in slowly, increase heat and allow to bubble before reducing heat to low. Cover and cook gently for 30 mins, stirring often

4. Remove bay leaves, stir and blend until smooth

5. Serve garnished.

Time: 20 mins | Serves 4

Calories: 1171	Carbs: 29.3g	Fibre: 10.8g	Protein: 157.3g

INGREDIENTS:

- ◆ 4 x 500g steaks
- ◆ 300g peeled carrots, sliced
- ◆ 300g frozen peas
- ◆ 300g broccoli, chopped
- ◆ 300g sliced green beans
- ◆ 4 tbsp butter
- ◆ Salt

PREPARATION:

1. Bring water to boil, lower heat and add vegetables. Cook for 5 to 10 mins

2. Rub salt onto steak

3. Meanwhile heat oil in heavy based frying pan to medium/ high heat and sear the steaks for 5 mins on each side, until done to personal taste

4. Serve with veggies

Time: 35 mins | Serves 4

Calories: 485	Carbs: 15g	Fibre: 4.4g	Protein: 25g

INGREDIENTS:

- ◆ 400g pack sausages
- ◆ 2 tbsp olive oil
- ◆ 2 finely chopped garlic cloves
- ◆ 1 finely chopped onion
- ◆ roughly sliced red bell pepper
- ◆ 200g lentils
- ◆ 300ml vegetable stock

PREPARATION:

1. Brown sausages for 4 mins in oil heated over medium heat. Drain on paper towel once removed

2. Cook onion, bell pepper and garlic over medium heat in 1 tbsp of oil for 4 mins until soft

3. Add lentils, stock and sausages to the pan, bring to boil. Simmer for 25 mins

4. Serve

Time: 30 mins | Serves 4

Calories: 339	Carbs: 33.3g	Fibre: 3.1g	Protein: 6.3g

INGREDIENTS:

- 400gcooked and drained brown rice,
- 8 eggs
- 1 onion
- 200g tinned tomatoes, finely chopped
- 1finely chopped green chilli
- 1 tbsp vegetable oil
- 1tsp turmeric powder
- 2 tsp finely chopped ginger
- 4 garlic cloves, finely chopped
- 250g diced celeriac
- coriander
- Salt to taste
- 1 tsp garam masala

PREPARATION:

1. Fry onion for 4-5 minutes until it turns brown, add garlic and ginger, and stir well

2. Add tomatoes, chilli, garam masala, turmeric powder, and salt to taste. Cook for further 3 mins. Add boiling water and simmer for $4\frac{7}{8}$ mins

3. Boil eggs and diced celeriac in medium-size saucepan for 7 mins, drain and peel and peel and halve eggs

4. Gently stir egg and celeriac into the curry, and cook for further 5 mins

5. Serve with brown rice, garnished with fresh coriander.

TIME: 20 MINS | SERVES 5

Calories: 550	Carbs: 17g	Fat: 50g	Protein: 4g

INGREDIENTS:

- ◆ 2 cups almond flour
- ◆ 1 tbsp coconut oil
- ◆ 8 tbsp butter, melted
- ◆ ¼ cup water
- ◆ 4 eggs
- ◆ 1 tsp baking powder
- ◆ 2 tbsp sweetener
- ◆ 1 tsp vanilla essence
- ◆ extra butter for griddle
- ◆ pinch salt

PREPARATION:

1. Blend all ingredients, mixing until fully combined.

2. Set one side for 5 mins.

3. Pour ⅓ cup portion into skillet/non-stick pan and cook over medium low heat until edges firm. Flip and cook other side for 1 min. These pancakes do not bubble up like traditional pancakes when cooked.

4. Serve hot.

TIME: 3 mins | SERVES 4

Calories: 60	Carbs: 13g	Fibre: 1g	Sugar: 9g	Protein: 1g

INGREDIENTS:

- ♦ 450g tinned garbanzo beans, rinsed and drained
- ♦ 400g tinned artichoke hearts, rinsed drained and quartered
- ♦ 450g tinned French-style green beans, drained
- ♦ ½ cup Italian salad dressing

PREPARATION:

1. Combine all ingredients, toss and serve chilled.

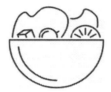

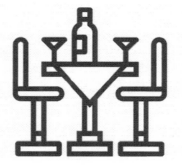

TIME: 25 MINS | SERVES 4

Calories: 281	Carbs: 11g	Fibre: 3g	Sugar: 6g	Protein: 30g

INGREDIENTS:

- ◆ 580g salmon fillet, divided into 4
- ◆ 1⅞ bell peppers, trimmed, halved and seeded
- ◆ 1 baby marrow, halved lengthwise
- ◆ 1 tbsp extra-virgin olive oil
- ◆ 1red onion
- ◆ ¼ cup basil, finely sliced
- ◆ 1 lemon, quartered
- ◆ If you want to use salt and pepper, do it

PREPARATION:

1. Preheat grill to med-high

2. Coat marrows, peppers and onion with oil and use the salt

3. Season salmon

4. Grill vegetables and salmon pieces, skin-side down. Turn veg once or twice, cooking for 4 to 5 mins per side.

5. Do not turn the salmon during 8 to 10 mins on grill, cooking until it flakes with a fork

6. Roughly chop the cooked vegetables and toss together

7. Serve the salmon with skin removed, alongside the vegetables, a lemon wedge, and garnished with basil.

TIME: 40 MINS | SERVES 2

Calories: 329	Carbs: 35g	Fibre: 2g	Sugar: 8g	Protein: 29g

INGREDIENTS:

- 1 cup potato gnocchi, drained after cooking
- 225g pork tenderloin, trimmed and sliced into 1.5cm slices
- 2 tsp canola oil
- 2 tbsp shallot, grated
- 1 tsp butter
- 3 tbsp lime juice
- 190g kale leaves
- 2 large cloves garlic, grated
- 2 tsp honey
- lime wedges

PREPARATION:

1. Drizzle and toss pork with lime juice, cover and set aside to marinate at room temperature for 15 mins. Drain

2. Cook pork in oil heated over medium-high heat for 2 mins on each side. Remove from skillet, cover with foil and keep warm

3. In the same skillet, melt butter and add shallot, kale, garlic, and cooked gnocchi. Stir occasionally while cooking for 5 to 8 mins

4. Drizzle with honey and toss to mix

5. Serve with lime wedges.

Time: 1hr 40 mins | Serves 8

| Calories: 272 | Carbs: 23g | Fibre: 6g | Protein: 24g |

INGREDIENTS:

- 900g pork loin roast
- 700g carrots, chopped
- 700g peeled parsnips, chopped
- 1 tsp honey
- 2 tsp fresh thyme
- 3 tbsp extra-virgin olive oil
- 1cup cider
- Chutney

PREPARATION:

1. Preheat oven to 401°F (201°C).

2. Toss carrots and parsnips with 2 tbsp oil, 1 tsp thyme, salt and pepper and spread evenly in roasting pan

3. Rub pork with remaining oil, thyme, salt and pepper and arrange fat-side up on top of vegetables

4. Cook in oven for 50 to 65 mins, stirring vegetables occasionally

5. Remove pork, tent with foil and put one side for15 mins

6. Stir honey into vegetables in a bowl

7. Heat roasting pan over two burners on high heat and add cider, scraping browned bits, for 3 to 5 mins

8. Serve the pork sliced, with the vegetables, sauce and chutney.

Calories: 290	Carbs: 40g	Fibre: 7g	Sugar: 7g	Protein: 9g

INGREDIENTS:

- ◆ 350g dried whole-grain pasta, cooked and drained
- ◆ 1⅞ red bell peppers, cleaned and halved lengthwise
- ◆ 1⅓ cups whole peeled plum tomatoes
- ◆ ½ cup whole toasted almonds
- ◆ 1 tbsp sherry vinegar
- ◆ 3 tbsp olive oil
- ◆ 1⅞ tbsp fresh Italian parsley, chopped
- ◆ 2 cloves garlic
- ◆ 1⅛ tbsp honey
- ◆ ½ tsp smoked paprika
- ◆ ¼ cup grated Parmesan

PREPARATION:

1. Preheat oven to 400°F (200°C) and lightly oil a baking sheet

2. Roast bell peppers with cut sides up, on baking sheet for 45 min. Remove, and cover them with cling wrap in a bowl. Set aside until cool enough to peel skin off

3. To prepare sauce, blend roasted peppers, tomatoes, almonds, oil, 2 tbsp parsley, sherry vinegar, honey, garlic, salt, and smoked paprika until nearly smooth

4. Boil sauce to boil and simmer for 20 mins

5. Serve pasta with sauce as you like it.

TIME: 4HRS 50 MINS | SERVES 2

Calories: 338	Carbs: 29g	Fibre: 3g	Sugar: 7g	Protein: 32g

INGREDIENTS:

- 900g pork shoulder roast, trimmed
- 1⅞ tsp chili powder
- 1 cup water
- ½ cup tomatillos, husked and chopped
- 2 tbsp finely chopped fresh jalapeño chile pepper
- 2 tbsp finely chopped onion
- 1⅛ tbsp fresh coriander, chopped
- 1⅛ tbsp lime juice
- 2 cloves garlic, grated
- 6 (6 inch) yellow corn tortillas, warmed
- 6 tbsp chopped fresh mango

PREPARATION:

1. Sprinkle pork with chili powder and seasoning. Cook in slow cooker with ½ cup water on low-heat setting for 9 to 10 hrs OR high-heat setting for 4½ to 5 hrs.

2. Remove when cooked and pull the pork using a fork

3. Prepare salsa verde by cooking tomatillos, onion, chile pepper, coriander, lime juice, garlic, pepper, salt and ½ cup water, stirring over medium heat for 15 mins.

4. Cool slightly and serve tortillas topped with shredded pork, salsa verde, and mango.

TIME: 25 MINS | SERVES 4

Calories: 161	Carbs: 7g	Fibre: 2g	Sugar: 4g	Protein: 21g

INGREDIENTS:

- ♦ 4 x 115g skinless fish fillets, ⅞ to 2cm thick
- ♦ 1 tbsp olive oil
- ♦ 1 can whole tomatoes, drained and chopped
- ♦ 2 cloves garlic, crushed
- ♦ 1 thinly sliced onion
- ♦ 2 tsp fresh thyme, chopped
- ♦ 8 Greek olives, pitted and halved
- ♦ 1 tsp capers, drained
- ♦ Fresh thyme sprigs

PREPARATION:

1. Line a broiler pan with foil and preheat broiler

2. Prepare sauce by cooking garlic and onion in oil in small saucepan for 5 mins heated over medium heat, until tender, stirring occasionally

3. Add tomatoes, thyme, capers, and olives, bring to boil and simmer uncovered for 10 mins

4. Broil fish for 4 to 6 mins/1cm thickness of fish, until you think it is done. Turn once if fillets are 2.5cm thick

5. Serve with sauce garnished with fresh thyme sprigs.

TIME: 20 MINS | SERVES 4

Calories: 156	Carbs: 29g	Fibre: 6g	Sugar: 4g	Protein: 6g

INGREDIENTS:

- ¼ cup fresh coriander, chopped
- 2 tbsp canola oil
- 3 tbsp lime juice
- 1¼ cups water
- pinch cayenne pepper
- 1½ tsp grated fresh ginger
- 1 425g tin black beans, rinsed and drained
- 1 medium red bell pepper, seeded and coarsely chopped
- 1 cup whole-wheat couscous
- 2 cups coarsely shredded fresh spinach
- ¼ cup thinly sliced scallions
- 1 medium mango, peeled, seeded, and chopped

PREPARATION:

1. Prepare dressing by whisking coriander, lime juice, oil, ginger, salt, and cayenne pepper together. Set aside

2. Bring water to boil in a medium saucepan, stir in couscous when off the heat, cover and set aside for 5 mins. Follow cooking instructions further

3. Meanwhile combine beans, bell pepper, spinach, scallions and mango, add couscous and reserved dressing. Toss to coat.

4. Serve immediately or refrigerate covered with plastic wrap/foil for up to 24 hours.

TIME: 45 MINS | SERVES 4

Calories: 245	Carbs: 13g	Fibre: 4g	Sugar:6g	Protein: 28g

INGREDIENTS:

- *Steak & Vegetables*
- 450g sirloin steak, 2cm thick
- 1⅞ cups cherry tomatoes
- 2⅛ baby marrows, halved lengthwise
- ½ tsp chili powder
- 1 red onion, sliced 1cm thick
- Non-stick spray
- *Chimichurri Sauce*
- ½ cup coriander
- 1 cup parsley
- 6 cloves garlic, minced
- ¼ cup white wine vinegar
- 1 tbsp olive oil
- 2 tbsp water
- Salt and Pepper

PREPARATION:

1. Trim steak and divide equally into four portions. Sprinkle with chili powder and salt.

2. Skewer tomatoes onto four metal skewers and coat lightly with non-stick spray

3. Use non-stick spray on baby marrow and onion slices and season vegetables with salt

4. Grill steak, tomato skewers and vegetable slices over medium coals until cooked, turning once, 14 - 18 mins for medium-rare; 18 - 22 mins for medium

5. Grill marrows and onion slices for 10 to 11 mins, turning often. Grill tomatoes for 4 to 5 mins, turning once until lightly charred

6. Blend parsley, coriander, water, garlic vinegar, salt, and black pepper and olive oil being careful not to puree

7. Serve steak sliced with grilled vegetable slices, tomatoes, and Chimichurri Sauce.

Time: 3hrs 20 mins | Serves 4

Calories: 317	Carbs: 43g	Fibre: 14g	Sugar: 4g	Protein: 24g

INGREDIENTS:

- ◆ 450g minced meat
- ◆ 1 chopped onion
- ◆ Not quite 3 cups mashed potatoes
- ◆ 450g mixed vegetables, frozen
- ◆ 305g tin tomato soup
- ◆ 1 cup dry brown lentils, rinsed and drained
- ◆ 400g tin beef broth
- ◆ 410g tin diced tomatoes, oregano, garlic and basil, not drained
- ◆ ¼ tsp red pepper

PREPARATION:

1. Brown meat and onion and drain off fat

2. Cook frozen vegetables, tomatoes, lentils, tomato soup, broth, red pepper and meat mixture in slow cooker for 6 to 8hrs on low-heat setting OR for 3 to 4hrs on high-heat setting

3. Serve over mashed potatoes.

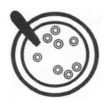

Time: 5hrs 10 min | Serves 4

| Calories: 251 | Carbs: 11g | Fibre: 0g | Sugar: 10g | Protein: 30g |

INGREDIENTS:

- ◆ 900g meaty chicken pieces, skinned
- ◆ 1 tbsp grated fresh ginger
- ◆ ½ cup freshly squeezed orange juice
- ◆ 1 tbsp olive oil
- ◆ ½ tsp ground coriander
- ◆ 1 tsp ground cumin
- ◆ 1 tsp paprika
- ◆ 2 tsp finely mushed orange peel
- ◆ 2 tbsp honey
- ◆ 2 tsp juice of orange
- ◆ Salt and pepper

PREPARATION:

1. Preheat oven to 377°F (191°C)

2. Place chicken in resealable plastic bag set in a deep dish

3. Prepare marinade by stirring together cup of orange juice, olive oil, cumin, ginger, paprika, coriander, pepper, and salt

4. Cover chicken with marinade and seal bag, turning to coat chicken. Marinate for 4 – 24 hrs in refrigerator, turning the bag occasionally.

5. Meanwhile, stir together orange peel, honey, and 2 tsp orange juice in a small bowl

6. Drain chicken and bake skin sides up, in shallow baking dish

for 45 to 55 mins, until done, brushing occasionally with honey mixture during final 10 mins

7. Serve

Time: 5hrs 20 mins | Serves 4

Calories: 340	Carbs: 34g	Fibre: 3g	Sugar: 4g	Protein: 35g

INGREDIENTS:

- ♦ 1.5kg beef stew meat, cubed into bite sizes
- ♦ 3 cups chopped onions
- ♦ 3 cloves garlic, minced
- ♦ 1 170g tin tomato paste
- ♦ 1½ cups coarsely chopped green sweet peppers
- ♦ 4 tsp paprika
- ♦ ½ cup water
- ♦ 5⅞ cups hot cooked noodles

PREPARATION:

1. Combine tomato paste, paprika, salt, water, and black pepper

2. Place sweet peppers onions, and garlic in slow cooker and top with meat. Pour tomato paste mixture over meat and cook for 10 to 12hrs on low-heat setting OR 5 to 6hrs on high-heat setting

3. Serve over noodles.

TIME: 40 MINS | SERVES 6

Calories: 345	Carbs: 37g	Fibre: 8g	Sugar: 7g	Protein: 13g

INGREDIENTS:

- ◆ 450g sweet potatoes, peeled and cubed
- ◆ 2 tbsp canola oil
- ◆ 4 tsp red curry paste
- ◆ 1½ cups diced onion
- ◆ 1 tbsp grated fresh ginger
- ◆ 1 tbsp grated garlic
- ◆ 1 grated serrano chile, seeds removed
- ◆ 1 cup coconut milk
- ◆ 3 cups water
- ◆ ¾ cup unsalted dry-roasted peanuts
- ◆ 425g tin white beans, rinsed
- ◆ ¼ cup unsalted roasted pumpkin seeds
- ◆ ¼ cup chopped fresh coriander
- ◆ 2 tbsp lime juice
- ◆ Lime wedges
- ◆ Salt & pepper

PREPARATION:

1. Cook onion in oil heated over medium-high heat in large pot, stirring often, for 4 mins until translucent. Add curry paste, garlic, ginger, and serrano, stirring for 1 min

2. Stir in sweet potatoes and water and bring to boil, simmering partially covered for 10 to 12 mins

3. Puree half the soup with coconut milk and peanuts in a blender, and return to the pot with remaining soup

4. Add beans, salt, and pepper, stir and heat

5. Stir in lime juice and coriander once off the heat

6. Serve with lime wedges and pumpkin seeds

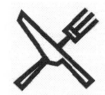

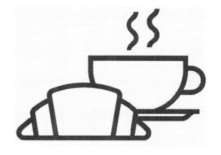

Time: 10 mins | Serves 8

Calories: 106	Carbs: 7g	Fibre: 2g	Sugar: 0g	Protein: 3g

INGREDIENTS:

- ◆ 425g tin chickpeas, drained and rinsed
- ◆ 2 tbsp extra virgin olive oil
- ◆ 1 clove chopped garlic
- ◆ ¼ cup tahini
- ◆ ½ tsp ground cumin
- ◆ 2 tbsp fresh lemon juice
- ◆ Salt

PREPARATION:

1. Blend chickpeas, tahini, oil, lemon juice, garlic, cumin, and salt until smooth

2. Use immediately or store refrigerated for up to 7 days.

Time: 7 mins | Serves 5 slices

Carbs: 24g	Fibre: 4g	Protein: 7g

Ingredients:

- ◆ 1 large sweet potato, sliced lengthwise into 7mm thick slices
- ◆ Suggested toppings: Dijon Mustard and smoked salmon

Preparation:

1. Toast sweet potato slices in toaster not on low and not on medium for 5 mins, until cooked through

2. Serve with preferred toppings or store in airtight glass container for up to a week.

Time: 15 mins | Yields 48 chips

Calories not given

INGREDIENTS:

- ♦ 6 tortillas
- ♦ 1 tbsp coconut oil, melted
- ♦ ¼ cup nutritional yeast
- ♦ 1 tsp onion powder
- ♦ 2 tsp paprika
- ♦ 1 ½ tsp chili powder
- ♦ ½ tsp coconut sugar
- ♦ ¼ tsp garlic powder
- ♦ 1 tsp salt

PREPARATION:

1. Preheat oven to 377°F (180°C). Spray non-stick spray on baking sheet

2. Get 8 chips from each tortilla by stacking them evenly, slicing half, and in half again, and then cutting the pieces in half

3. Layer on the baking sheet and lightly brush both sides with the oil

4. Combine nutritional yeast, paprika, onion powder, chili powder, salt, coconut sugar, and garlic powder

5. Sprinkle tortillas with the mixture. Bake until lightly browned and crispy, 8 to 10 mins. Let rest for 5 mins before serving.

Non given

INGREDIENTS:

- ◆ 2 tins canned chickpeas, rinsed and drained
- ◆ 1 ½ tsp extra-virgin olive oil
- ◆ ½ tsp each ground cumin and ground coriander
- ◆ ¼ tsp each ground red pepper and ground black pepper

PREPARATION:

1. Preheat the oven to 401°F (201°C). Spray baking sheet with non-stick spray

2. Toss the chickpeas, oil, coriander, cumin, red pepper and black pepper in a small bowl

3. Bake chickpeas spread over baking sheet for 31 to 40 mins, until golden and crisp.

TIME: 12HRS 22 | IN YIELDS 5

Calories: 144	Carbs: 17g	Fibre: 3g	Protein: 5.6g

INGREDIENTS:

- ◆ 1 cup rolled oats
- ◆ 5 tbsp black lentils
- ◆ 1½ cups water
- ◆ 5 tsp ghee
- ◆ Salt

PREPARATION:

1. Blend oats and lentils to a smooth powder, add water and blend further until smooth

2. Transfer to deep bowl, cover and set aside to ferment for approximately 11hrs, then add salt and mix very well

3. Pour ladle full of batter into heated non-stick pan or non-stick griddle in 175mm diameter circle

4. Smear with ghee and crisp over high heat. Fold into semi-circle and repeat for remaining dosas

5. Serve immediately

Time: 22 mins | Serves 6

Calories: 336	Carbs: 36.9g	Fibre: 13.2g	Sugar: 1.3g	Protein: 11.9g

INGREDIENTS:

- 200g 85% dark chocolate
- 4 eggs
- 1 egg yolk
- 60g artificial sweetener
- 120g butter
- 30g buckwheat flour
- ⅓ cup roasted and salted pistachios, chopped
- ¼ cup (60ml) coconut milk
- 30g cornflour

PREPARATION:

1. Preheat oven to 390°F (200°C). Grease 6 ramekins

2. Melt the chocolate and butter in a saucepan stirring constantly over medium heat and then set one side

3. Whisk eggs, sweetener and egg yolk until smooth, add buckwheat flour and corn flour using wooden spoon

4. Warm coconut milk over medium heat until it bubbles on side of saucepan. Remove from heat for before pouring hot milk slowly onto egg mixture, whisking vigorously, waiting a minute after removing from heat

5. Whisk in the melted chocolate and butter to a smooth chocolate batter consistency

6. Fill 6 ramekins with chocolate cake batter and bake for 12 to 15 mins, until a light crust forms

7. Avoid over-baking as the heart of the cakes must be runny. Serve immediately.

Non given

INGREDIENTS:

- 3 eggs
- 75g unsalted butter, melted and cooled
- 40g artificial sweetener
- 250ml milk
- 1 tsp vanilla extract
- 375g plain flour
- 2 tsp baking powder
- 250g fresh/frozen blueberries
- 30g brown sugar substitute
- 95g plain flour
- 2 tsp ground cinnamon
- 115g unsalted butter, softened

PREPARATION:

1. Preheat oven to 390°F (200°C). Grease and flour a 33 x 23 baking pan

2. Stir together melted butter, milk, eggs, vanilla and sugar substitute

3. Mix together 375g flour and baking powder and blend into wet ingredients. Fold in the blueberries and spread evenly in prepared tin

4. Combine brown sugar substitute, 95g flour and cinnamon

and stir in softened butter using a fork until crumbly. Sprinkle over top of cake and bake for 35 to 40 mins

5. Best served warm.

Time: 80 mins | Serves 12

Calories: 241	Carbs: 24g	Fat: 9g	Protein: 17g

INGREDIENTS:

- ◆ 225g self-raising flour
- ◆ ½ tsp baking powder
- ◆ 5 tbsp canola oil
- ◆ 140g agave syrup
- ◆ 1 tsp ground cinnamon
- ◆ 1 apple, peeled, cored and diced
- ◆ 85g diced dried apricots
- ◆ 140g finely grated carrot
- ◆ 50g pumpkin seeds
- ◆ grated zest of 1 orange + 5 tbsp juice
- ◆ icing sugar for dusting

PREPARATION:

1. Preheat oven to 370°F (180°C). Grease a cake tin

2. Mix flour, baking powder and cinnamon in a large bowl, add orange juice, agave syrup and oil and stir well. Stir in grated carrot, apple, orange zest, and apricots until well mixed.

3. Spoon into prepared tin and bake for 50 mins.

TIME: 40 MINS | SERVES 12 slices

Calories: 216	Carbs: 12.7g	Fibre: 5.3g	Sugar: 4.7g	Protein: 5.8g

INGREDIENTS:

- *Walnuts Almond Crust*
- 1 egg
- 1⅛ cup almond meal
- 1 cup walnuts
- 6 tbsp coconut flour
- ¼ cup extra virgin coconut oil
- 4 tbsp artificial sweetener
- *Blueberry filling*
- 3 cup frozen blueberries
- 1/3 cup chia seeds
- 3 tbsp lukewarm water
- 1 tsp vanilla extract
- 4 tbsp artificial sweetener

PREPARATION:

1. Preheat oven to 370°F (180°C). Cover work surface with cling wrap

2. Using 'S' blade attachment, combine all the crust ingredients at medium speed for 1 min, until mixture comes together to form a ball

3. Transfer the dough to prepared surface covered and set aside a quarter of the dough to use for decorating

4. Place cling wrap over dough, and roll dough as for a regular

pie crust to fit the pie dish. Remove the top layer of cling wrap and flip the crust into the pie dish. Push the dough until it fits the dish perfectly.

5. Bake for 15 to 20 mins, until crispy and golden

6. Prepare filling by stirring together lukewarm water and chia seeds. Set aside for 2 mins for seeds to absorb the water, stirring occasionally

7. Warm blueberries and sweetener in a covered saucepan over medium heat until bubbles start to form on the side. Stir in soaked chia seeds and simmer for 4 to 8 mins, until jelly-like

8. Pour jam onto the prepared crust. Bake for 10 mins and let cool before unmoulding.

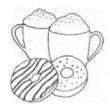

TIME: 15 MINS | SERVES 4

Calories: 297	Carbs: 3.7g	Sugar: 0.3g	Protein: 8.6g

INGREDIENTS:

- ◆ 1 tsp vanilla extract
- ◆ 2 cups milk
- ◆ 4 egg yolks
- ◆ 1 cup artificial sweetener
- ◆ *Poached Meringue*
- ◆ ½ cup to ⅔ cup dark chocolate chips
- ◆ 4 egg whites
- ◆ 2 tbsp artificial sweetener
- ◆ *Topping*
- ◆ ¼ cup raspberries
- ◆ 2 tbsp sliced almonds

PREPARATION:

1. Bring milk and vanilla extract to boil. Seat one side after removing from heat

2. Add sweetener to egg yolk and beat at medium/high speed for 30/45 secs until lighter and fluffy. Stir lukewarm vanilla milk mixture into egg yolk mixture and return to saucepan, stirring for 10 mins over low/medium heat. Remove from heat, cool and refrigerate for 2-3 hrs

3. For the meringue, beat egg white for 45 seconds at medium/ high speed, until starting to firm

4. Add sweetener. Beat until a stiff peaks form. Set one side

5. Bring 1000ml water to boil in a saucepan and simmer. Plunge a scoop of meringue mixture into the water and poach for 30 seconds. Remove and refrigerate

6. To serve divide vanilla custard into 4 serving bowls, top with cooled meringue and drizzle with melted chocolate, sliced almonds or berries.

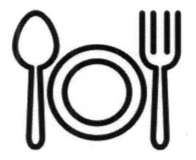

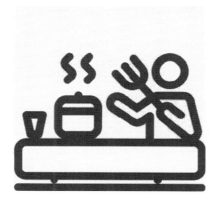

The idea of entertaining at home or eating out should not be overwhelming for a diabetic or anyone catering for a diabetic guest. Many restaurants will accommodate you, knowing that you have specific dietary requirements. When dining out, the important aspects are calories and portion sizes, and these suggestions may be helpful:

- The Diabetes Plate Method comes in particularly useful here, as outlined in the opening of this book.

- Alcohol can affect blood sugar and due cognisance should be paid accordingly. The guidelines for safe alcohol consumption seems to be one drink a day with a meal for diabetic women or two for men. One drink is 350ml serving of beer, 150ml serving of wine, or 45ml of distilled spirits, such as vodka or whiskey.

- Italian, Chinese, Thai and Indian restaurants typically serve foods higher in carbs, so portion sizes must be carefully monitored when dining at any of these establishments.

ᛥ Opt for meat, fish or chicken.

ᛥ Tomato and vegetable-based sauces are better options than creamy or cheese-based sauces. Request that sauce be served on the side

ᛥ Salads should be ordered without creamy dressings. Ask for a balsamic vinegar, vinaigrette, or lemon juice dressing to be served on the side.

ᛥ Order food grilled, roasted or baked instead of battered, fried, or creamy.

ᛥ Dessert options to go for include sorbets or fruit-based treats over pastries and cakes or cheese and biscuits.

When catering for diabetics at home, especially for holiday festivities, it is very easy to substitute suitable foods without any problems. This should give you some ideas:

ᛥ *Water*

Set the table with a jug of water, either plain or infused with lemon or cucumber and make sure to have unsweetened iced tea as an option.

ᛥ *Sides*

On the subject of setting the table, make sure to offer whole grain dinner rolls as a side dish.

ᛥ *Snacks*

To keep blood sugar levels stable, diabetics need to eat more often. For this reason, it's a good idea to have diabetic-friendly snacks available before the meal is served, to tide the guests over. Winners include vegetable crudités, hummus dips, cocktail onions, olives and gherkins.

◌ *Substitute solid fats with liquid fats*

- Limit saturated fats and avoid trans fats, so substitute solid fat (butter, lard, hydrogenated shortening) with trans-fat free margarine, spreads, or shortening.

- Liquid fats can be healthy in moderation (olive, canola, corn, and grape seed).

◌ *Manage the carbohydrates*

- Choose carbs that provide fibre and long-lasting energy.

- Substitute white rice, white flour, and refined grains with brown rice, whole wheat flour, whole-grain flours/grain products and ground nuts like hazelnut or almond meal.

◌ *Low and Medium-GI vegetable dishes*

Include sweet potatoes along with regular potato options and have green beans, broccoli, tomatoes, or eggplant.

◌ *Sugar*

Substitute or cut back on sugar without impeding the taste of food by using sweeteners intended for baking.

◌ *Flavour Experimenting.*

- Sugar, salt, and fat can be substituted with healthy options without losing the taste. Mustards, vinegars (sherry/

balsamic), herbs, and spices (cinnamon, cardamom, nutmeg) have health benefits, some of which even lowering blood sugar levels

- Canned and frozen foods typically contain more salt than fresh foods

- Salt in a recipe is really replaceable unless the recipe calls for yeast too, which requires salt for rising. The best option is not to cook with salt at all, only having it as an option on the table

- Opt for unsalted nuts over salted.

∂ *Use low-fat dairy options*

- Substitute full-cream milk or half-and-half with 1%, skim milk, non-fat half-and-half, or condensed skim milk.

- Substitute sour cream with buttermilk, low-fat/non-fat plain yogurt, or low-fat cottage cheese

- For sauces, substitute cream/full-cream milk with skim milk and corn starch.

∂ *Cut down on fat*

- Cut back fat ingredients in recipes by 25% to 33%

- Substitute fats in baked goods with mashed bananas or applesauce

- Substitute chocolate/chocolate chips with cocoa powder or fewer mini-chocolate chips

- Skim fat off soups or stew before serving.

ଡ Dessert

- Place fresh fruit on the table after the meal so that your diabetic guests can indulge on the healthy side.

Time: 5hrs | Serves 8

Calories: 256	Carbs: 23g	Fibre: 4g	Sugar: 5g	Protein: 34g

INGREDIENTS:

- 1 tsp dried rosemary, crushed
- ¼ tsp dried thyme, crushed
- ¼ tsp garlic powder
- 1 x 1.25 – 1.5kg turkey breast half, bone-in and skinned
- 1 tbsp vegetable oil1
- 115g new potatoes, halved
- 8 carrots, peeled and cut into 4 to 6cm lengths
- 1 onion, cut into wedges
- ¼ cup flour
- 125ml chicken broth
- Ground pepper and salt

PREPARATION:

1. Rub turkey breast with a mix of rosemary, salt, garlic powder, thyme and pepper

2. Brown turkey breast in hot oil over medium heat on all sides in large skillet

3. Place potatoes, carrots, onion and ¼ cup broth in slow cooker coated with non-stick spray and top with turkey. Cover and cook on low for 9 hrs OR on high for 4½ hours. Remove, cover loosely with foil and set aside for 15 mins

4. Meanwhile, move vegetables to a serving platter and keep warm

5. Prepare gravy by straining cooking liquid into a measuring jug to which enough broth to equal 1¾ cups is to be added

6. Whisk ¼ cup cold broth and flour together until smooth in a medium saucepan and then whisk in remaining broth mix. Stir over medium heat until bubbly and thickened, cook for further minute and add pepper to taste

7. Remove turkey from bone, slice and serve with vegetables and gravy.

TIME: **75** MINS | SERVES **4**

Calories: 429	Carbs: 89.5g	Fibre: 15.8g	Protein: 14.2g

INGREDIENTS:

- 1 cup quinoa, dry
- 2 – 3 cups butternut, diced
- 1½ cups chickpeas, cooked
- ½ cup chopped onion
- ½ cup raisins
- 1 juiced lime
- 2 tbsp balsamic vinegar
- ½ tsp cumin
- 1 clove garlic
- 2 dates, pitted

PREPARATION:

1. Preheat oven to 375ºF (180°C). Line baking sheet

2. Bake butternut for an hour, turning once

3. Meanwhile cook the quinoa as directed, remove from heat and stir in chickpeas, onion, and raisins and then the cooked butternut

4. Make the dressing by blending balsamic vinegar, lime juice, dates, garlic, and cumin

5. To serve, our dressing over quinoa and enjoy over greens of your choice.

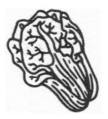

Time: 36 mins | Serves 4

Calories: 276	Carbs: 63.1g	Fibre: 4.7g	Sugar: 2.4g	Protein: 7.7g

INGREDIENTS:

- ◆ 1.4kg (9 cups) peeled potatoes, chopped into bite sized chunks
- ◆ 2 tsp garlic salt
- ◆ 1 tsp onion salt
- ◆ ¼ cup chopped chives/onions/parsley to garnish

PREPARATION:

1. Cover potatoes with water in a soup pot and add garlic salt and onion salt. Bring to boil uncovered and cook for 15 to 20 mins

2. Drain potatoes and reserve 250ml of cooking water

3. Beat potatoes on low speed, gradually adding reserved water to desired consistency.

4. Garnish as required. Serve with creamy Mushroom Gravy (Recipe below)

TIME: 21 MINS | YIELDS 4 CUPS

Calories: 57	Carbs: 7.9g	Fibre: 1.6g	Sugar: 3.1g	Protein: 2.5g

INGREDIENTS:

- 2½ cups chopped white mushrooms
- 2 cups water
- 1 tsp poultry seasoning
- 2 tsp finely chopped garlic
- ¼ cup raw unsalted cashews
- 1 cup onion, chopped
- ½ cup thinly sliced carrot
- ½ cup sliced celery
- Ground black pepper

PREPARATION:

1. Blend water and cashews and set one side for 15 mins or longer

2. Heat 1 tbsp water in saucepan over medium-high heat until it starts to sputter. Add mushrooms, carrots, celery, and onions, stir while cooking for 2 to 3 mins

3. Add garlic and poultry seasoning and stir for further 2 to 3 mins

4. Blend cooked vegetables with water and cashew mixture until very smooth, gradually adding water if necessary

5. Simmer the gravy in saucepan over medium-low heat to

heat through. Serve seasoned to taste with black pepper over mashed potatoes (recipe above) or dish of choice.

Time: 35 mins | Makes 1 pie

Calories: 134	Carbs: 16.5g	Fibre: 2.8g	Sugar: 6.6g	Protein: 2.6g

INGREDIENTS:

- 1¼ cups rolled oats
- ½ cup raw unsalted pecans
- ½ tsp cinnamon
- 70g pitted dates, chopped
- 1½ tbsp milk

PREPARATION:

1. Preheat the oven to 377 °F and prepare a20 x 20 x 5 cm pie pan

2. Blend oats, pecans, and cinnamon to a coarse flour consistency, add dates and blend for a minute until it clumps. Blend in milk until mixture balls up into dough

3. Form ball of dough on flat surface/parchment paper and flatten ball with your hands. Cover with parchment paper and use a rolling pin to roll into a circle about 3mm thick and a little bigger than the upper edge of the pie pan

4. Peel the top parchment paper off, invert the crust onto the pie pan and remove the remaining parchment paper. Lightly press the crust into the pan and trim away overhangs

5. Cover with foil, place on baking sheet and bake for 10 mins, until edges are lightly browned.

DISCLAIMER

This book is intended to be informative and helpful and contains the opinions and ideas of the author. The author intends to teach in an entertaining manner. Some recipes may not suit all readers. Use this book and implement the guides and recipes at your own will, taking responsibility and risk where it falls. This work with all its contents, does not guarantee correctness, completion, quality or correctness of the provided information. Misinformation or misprints cannot be completely eliminated.

LEGAL NOTICE

Made in the USA
Middletown, DE
21 January 2020